Magnesium Trace Mineral: Top 18 Benefits Of Magnesium And Why You Should Take It

All rights Reserved. No part of this publication or the information in it may be quoted from or reproduced in any form by means such as printing, scanning, photocopying or otherwise without prior written permission of the copyright holder.

Disclaimer and Terms of Use: Effort has been made to ensure that the information in this book is accurate and complete, however, the author and the publisher do not warrant the accuracy of the information, text and graphics contained within the book due to the rapidly changing nature of science, research, known and unknown facts and internet. The Author and the publisher do not hold any responsibility for errors, omissions or contrary interpretation of the subject matter herein. This book is presented solely for motivational and informational purposes only.

Table of Contents

Introduction

Magnesium is a mineral which is naturally present in various foods. It is present in abundant quantities in the human body. This mineral works as a cofactor along with more than 300 enzymes in our body and regulate the various biochemical reactions happening inside our system. An adult human body contains approximately 25 g magnesium and about 50 to 60 % is present in the bones and the rest of it is present in soft tissue. There are many sources of magnesium such as food, water, dietary supplements, medicines, etc. Our body absorbs about 30 to 40 % of the magnesium we consume. Magnesium deficiency is commonly seen elderly people and in African Americans. Athletes use this mineral to increase their energy levels and endurance. In older adults, the dietary intake of magnesium is lower compared to the younger adult. The absorption of Magnesium from gut decreases and renal excretion of magnesium increases with age.

One of the most important nutrients needed for a human body to function properly and disease free is magnesium. Be it sleep, fatigue, stress problems, abdominal fat, proper brain behavior, lean body compositor and many more, everything needs magnesium to function properly. It will also help in the production of testosterone, sensitivity of insulin, proper regulation for sympathetic nervous system, absorption of excess calcium in the blood, and regulates as many as 300 essential biochemical reactions. Magnesium that you get from the food that you take is more than sufficient or your body. But, in most cases, people do not take the required quantities of magnesium rich foods everyday and hence have to depend on magnesium supplementation to maintain a healthy and sound body. Magnesium is also lost from the body through alcohol, black tea, coffee, calcium supplements and pharmaceutical drugs.

An Important Trace Element

Magnesium is considered as an important trace element which is needed for the proper functioning of our body. Magnesium is needed for the synthesis of proteins, proper functioning of muscles and nerves, controlling the blood glucose level and for controlling the blood pressure level. Various energy producing and releasing cycles in our body such as Glycolysis, oxidative Phosphorylation requires the presence of magnesium in the body. Magnesium plays an important role in the proper structural development of the bones in our body. It is also necessary for the synthesis of nucleic acids such as DNA and RNA in our body. Transport of elements such as calcium and potassium across the cell membranes are regulated by the presence of magnesium. This is very important for maintaining the heart rhythm, conduction of nerve impulses in the body and for the contraction of muscles. Magnesium neutralizes the stomach acid and help in the movement of the stool through our intestine. It is effective in treating skin infections and wound healing. The level of the magnesium in our body is controlled by the kidneys. Our kidney excretes about 120 mg of magnesium through urine every day. When, the amount of Magnesium decreases in the body, the excretion of magnesium from the body through urine decrease. The recommended dietary allowance of magnesium depends on the age and sex of the person.

Recommended Daily Dose

These recommended daily requirements of magnesium in people of different age are

Children:

- 1 - 3 years old: 80 milligrams

- 4 - 8 years old: 130 milligrams

- 9 - 13 years old: 240 milligrams

- 14 - 18 years old (boys): 410 milligrams

- 14 - 18 years old (girls): 360 milligrams

Adults:

- Adult females: 310 - 320 milligrams

- Adult males: 400 - 420 milligrams

- Women during Pregnancy period: 350 - 400 milligrams

- Breastfeeding women: 310 - 360 milligrams

Food As A Source Of Magnesium

There are many animal and plant food sources of magnesium. Food derived from plants such as green leafy vegetables, legumes, nuts, whole grains, fruits and food from animal sources such as milk, chicken, fish, beef etc are rich sources of magnesium. Foods which are rich in dietary fibers such as spinach, almonds, black beans, avocado, breakfast cereals, oatmeal, banana, apple, carrot, raisins, and potato are high sources of the mineral.

Dietary Supplements As The Source

The dietary supplements of magnesium are available in different forms. The ability of the human body to absorb magnesium from these supplements vary. It is better to select supplements which are easily soluble in liquids so that they get absorbed well by the body. According to studies, magnesium in the form of aspartate, lactate, chloride and citrate is more absorbable than other forms. It is better to get magnesium in the natural form as present in food items rather than opting for supplements. If you are planning to take magnesium supplements, it is better to consult your doctor before that.

Medicines As The Source

Many of the medicines we consume such as laxatives, medicines for heartburn etc contain magnesium in the elemental form. Even though you are ingesting high doses of magnesium when you are taking laxatives, some of the magnesium will not get absorbed into the system due to the laxative effect of the medicine.

Deficiency Of Magnesium

Magnesium is the fourth most abundant mineral found in human body, however the deficiency of magnesium occurs in certain people. The causes of low magnesium level in the body are due to

- Excess use of caffeine

- Consumption of alcohol

- Excess use of sugar

- Regular consumption of processed food

- Consumption of fruits and vegetables produced from magnesium depleted soil

- Consumption of foods rich in phytic acid.

In some people only reduced absorption of magnesium occurs due to conditions such as

- Low level of calcium in blood

- Burns

- Use of certain medications

- Malabsorption of nutrients from intestinal tract

- After a surgery

Symptoms Of Deficiency Of Magnesium

The early symptoms of mild deficiency of magnesium in our body include

- Anorexia
- Poor memory
- Reduced ability to concentrate
- Fatigue or unusual tiredness
- Insomnia or lack of sleep
- Muscle twitching
- Infertility or PMS
- Reduced ability to learn
- Irritability
- Headaches
- Palpitation or hear flutter
- Lack of appetite
- Allergies and sensitivities
- Gut disorder

- Thyroid problems

- Insulin resistance

If you have five or more of the above symptoms you may have to go for magnesium supplementation.

The Symptoms For Moderate To High Deficiency Are

- Changes in heart function

- Rapid heart beat

- Numbness

- Continued muscle contraction

- Hallucinations

- Tingling sensation

When you have a deficiency of magnesium deficiency it will be difficult to raise the level of magnesium in your body by diet alone. You may need supplements in the appropriate forms to improve the condition.

Methods Of Supplementation

Magnesium can be supplemented for those having a deficiency of the mineral in the body. The different methods of supplementation are

- In powder form- You can use magnesium in the powder form and you can vary the dose according to the symptoms exhibited by the body.

- In liquid form- Magnesium in an ionic liquid form can be easily absorbed by the body when added to foods and drinks that are taken by a person.

- In transdermal oil form- magnesium when present in oil form can be applied to the skin for absorption. This is the best method to supplement magnesium as it is very effective, especially for people with severe deficiency of the mineral or people having a damaged digestive tract.

Health Risk from Magnesium

In healthy individuals excess intake of magnesium does not pose any health risk as their kidneys will eliminate the excess magnesium through urine. The high level of magnesium resulting from the consumption of medicines and dietary supplements may result in diarrhea, nausea and abdominal cramps. The symptoms of magnesium toxicity include hypotension, depression, facial flushing, nausea, vomiting, lethargy, Irregular heartbeat, difficulty in breathing. In people with impaired kidney function the risk of magnesium toxicity is more as the body will not be able to effectively remove the excess magnesium present in the body.

1. Better Sleep And Improves Endurance

Magnesium offers a calming effect on the nervous system and is very helpful to treat a lot of health problems. It is one of the best minerals that you can think of for treating insomnia. Lack of magnesium in the body has an adverse effect on the electrical activity of the brain and this will result in frequent awakenings as well as disturbed sleep at nights. It has been proven that taking magnesium supplements and adding magnesium rich foods has helped to reduce stress in people and allow them to relax. In fact, lower magnesium levels are also associated with greater body mass index. You will also experience elevated heart beat and response during exercise when you are low on magnesium. Hence, it is important for you to take adequate amount of magnesium rich foods that will help in de-stressing you and to make sure that you sleep peacefully at night without any distractions.

2. Builds Muscles

If you are looking to build your body and to improve the testosterone levels in your body, then you need adequate amounts of magnesium. It will help in boosting your metabolism and thereby you will be able to tone your body muscles. There have been tests conducted on athletes that proved that people who have taken adequate amounts of magnesium showed the greatest increase in the testosterone levels when training. It also helps in increasing the performance levels of a person.

3. Prevents Osteoporosis

Calcium is very important for healthy bones. But, without the adequate amounts of magnesium, the bones will not be healthy. It has been studied that decrease in magnesium levels has resulted in reduced bone strength, poor development of bones as well as decreased bone volume. Magnesium will help in releasing calcitonin hormone which is helpful in preserving the structure of the bone and will draw the calcium from the blood and give it to the bones. It is important for you to take adequate magnesium rich minerals that will help in improving your bone mineral density and keep your bones fit and healthy for a long time.

4. Lowers Risk Of Hypertension

Magnesium is found to be an excellent source that will help to lower blood pressure and to reduce the risk of hypertension. It will help in de-stressing a person and to relax him, thereby reducing the risk of increasing the blood pressure. Studies have shown that people who took 300 mg of magnesium supplements on a daily basis for three months showed greater reduction in the blood pressure levels. The systolic pressure was found to be decreased by 20 points and the diastolic pressure was found to fall by 10 points. A reduction in about 20 points means that the risk of getting a stroke or developing a heart disease is reduced by half. So, you need to take diets that are rich in magnesium and dietary fiber to stay clear from high blood pressure.

5. Improves Functioning Of The Brain

The brain electrical activity is greatly increased when you take required quantities of magnesium every day in the form of supplements or through magnesium rich foods. Magnesium will help in boosting memory and thereby help in elevated memory functions. It helps to increase the learning and memorizing capacity in students. If you are a person suffering from chronic low mood, then magnesium is the right supplement that will help in making your brain work better.

6. Reduces Body Inflammations

Inflammation of the body does not just prevent you from doing rigorous workouts, but also results in diabetes, Alzheimer's disease and heart disease. Magnesium deficiency will increase the inflammations in the body that will result in affecting blood vessels and cause cardiovascular inflammation which will result in heart disease. It will also decrease lipid metabolism and will impact the health of the arteries thereby resulting in atherosclerosis. It has been proved that adding magnesium of 365 mg to a diet helped in reducing the exercise induced chest pain. So, consuming magnesium on a daily basis will help you to have a healthy heart.

7. Prevents Diabetes

If you have low magnesium levels in your body, then it is very difficult for you to lose body fat as you will feel lower body metabolism. In fact, you will also be experiencing a decrease in insulin sensitivity. You will also be experiencing slower recovery after a workout session if you have lower levels of magnesium in your body. It is important for you to take care of your diabetes problems properly or else you will tend to lose a lot of magnesium in your body and this will magnify your health problem. Your kidneys will not be able to retain magnesium levels during hyperglycemia, which will result in you suffering from diabetes. If you would like to enjoy a lean body, then you need to take in adequate amounts of magnesium that your body needs daily. Taking in daily magnesium supplements and magnesium rich foods will help in improving the overall glucose metabolism in your body and help in boosting glucose transport.

8. Reduces Digestive Related Problems

If you have adequate intake of magnesium every day, then you will be experiencing 2 to 3 normal and soft bowel movements every day. People who are surfing from lower magnesium levels will experience harder bowel movement once in the space of two days. The lower levels of magnesium will also support certain symptoms like: irritability, insomnia, constipation, fatigue, poor mental function and muscle cramps. If there are higher levels of magnesium in your body, then you will not have any digestion problems and will enjoy a very healthy gastrointestinal tract. Hence, it will also help in reducing the risk of colon cancer and diabetes problems. You will not experience constipation problems if you take in good quantities of magnesium every day.

9. Prevents Metabolic Syndrome

Pregnant women suffer from low levels of metabolism, which might even result in them carrying diabetes and also seeing metabolic syndrome in the child after birth. It will result in an inflammatory condition that will increase oxidative stress and inflammation in the child. It is very important for pregnant women to maintain the required levels of magnesium in their body by taking magnesium supplements as prescribed by the doctors as well as eating magnesium rich foods.

10. Detoxifying Cortisol

It is necessary to lower your cortisol levels and it is possible to a great extent within the help of magnesium. If you do not take in the necessary magnesium on a daily basis, then you will feel de-stressed due to cortisol release. If you take adequate quantities of magnesium, then the magnesium will affect the release of norepinephrine which affects the sympathetic nervous system. With magnesium, you will be able to detoxify the cortisol levels and enjoy a stress free and relaxed state of mind.

11. Reduces Asthma

Magnesium has a lot of health benefits and one of the promising benefits is that it will help in treating asthma attacks. It will help in relaxing and smoothening the bronchial muscle in the same fashion as it does on the blood vessels. It has the ability to block the excess calcium as it works effectively on calcium channels across the cellular membranes. It has been proven that magnesium is useful in treating patients with severe acute asthma. It will help in boosting the expiratory flow rates and also will ensure proper breathing.

12. Supports Protein Synthesis

Magnesium helps in enabling the enzyme function of the body and hence it helps in boosting protein synthesis. It is important for you to take magnesium supplements when you carry out resistance exercise as it helps in making you stronger. It will help in muscle development and is part of every diet that any sportsperson or athletes take. It will help in easily gaining muscle mass and boost significant strength to the body during strength training. It is absolutely necessary for you to take adequate amounts of magnesium rich foods and supplements to enjoy healthy muscle development.

13.   Decreases ADHD

ADHD (attention deficit hyperactivity disorder) is a behavioral disorder that is seen very common in children and it normally starts during early stages of childhood. One of the main reasons for ADHD in children is lack of magnesium in the body. Even people of all ages can be affected by this behavioral disorder, but it is more commonly seen in children. It becomes very difficult for a child with ADHD to concentrate on the job or task at hand and gets always distracted. Children as well as adults suffering from ADHD find it very difficult to the physical activity that they carry out for certain works. It makes a person restless and impulsive. Taking adequate amounts of magnesium has proven to lower the ADHD problems in children and adults. Regular intake of magnesium supplements and magnesium rich foods helps in increasing the attention span of the person and it will offer calming and soothing effects on the person. It will also help in improving the activity of the brain.

14.　　Reduces Abdominal Obesity

Most of the people have fat deposits around their waist area. One of the most common areas that get accumulated by fat deposits is the waist and it is more commonly seen in people who do long hours of white collar jobs. Lack of magnesium levels in the body will result in increased waist circumference and increase in the fat deposits around the abdominal area. Magnesium plays an important role in weight management as it helps to regulate glucose levels and also improve the HDL cholesterol levels in the body. It is also a very powerful source that will stimulate protein synthesis and will also help in active body metabolism that will help to burn the fat easily. Magnesium is also found to be very effective treating people with excess obesity. It is very effective in treating metabolic syndrome and low grade inflammation in obese people and thereby will aid in reducing the weight of a person. Increase in the cortisol levels lead to high abdominal fat levels and with regular use of magnesium supplements and magnesium rich foods, the cortisol levels are greatly reduced. Taking magnesium in adequate levels will help in treating obesity and will also help a person to enjoy lean body composition.

15.   Treats Preeclampsia

Pregnancy induced hypertension or Preeclampsia is a condition that affects a lot of pregnant women in their later stages. Regular dose of magnesium supplements will help in preventing the progression of preeclampsia as well as eclamptic seizures that come along with preeclampsia. The progression of preeclampsia to eclampsia is prevented completely by taking adequate amounts of magnesium during pregnancy. The reduction of the dangerous hypertension problems by magnesium is because magnesium acts as a calcium antagonist. Magnesium also assists the release of prostaglandins which will reduce inflammation of the blood vessels and control blood pressures.

16.   Treats Migraine Headaches

It has been thoroughly researched and found out that Magnesium helps in treating as well as preventing migraines. It is ideal for people suffering from migraines and acute headaches to add regular dosages of magnesium supplements in their diet to get rid of migraine problems. Treatment through oral magnesium is found to be very effective in preventing and treating minor migraines. Any person suffering from serious or acute migraine headaches, then intravenous magnesium treat will help in effectively reducing migraine problems.

17. Reduces Depression

If you are suffering from chronic or major depression problems, then you need to take in adequate amounts of magnesium supplementation. It is proven clinically to be very effective in treating depression in men and women. People who are suffering from depression and mental instability are prone to suicides and suicide attempts. So, it is important for you to remain depression free and the best way is to increase the intake of magnesium rich foods and to include magnesium supplementation in your diet.

18. Other Magnesium Benefits

Some of the other benefits that you will get by taking in magnesium supplementation and magnesium rich diet on a daily basis are as follows.

- Magnesium is a very good electrolyte that will help in staying dehydrated for a long time as it supports proper hydration.

- Magnesium is needed for proper functioning of the enzymes in your body.

- Magnesium helps in maintaining the pH balance of the body. It will also help in reducing lactic acid in the body.

- Magnesium is necessary for mineralizing your teeth. If your body is devoid of magnesium, then your teeth will be damaged due to imbalance of calcium and phosphorus in the saliva.

- It also helps in reducing period pains and prevention of stroke and heart disease.

- It will also help in offering yo0u better flexibility by tightening your muscles and allow them to relax properly so that you do not suffer from muscle cramps.

- Magnesium helps in the production of adenosine triphosphate (ATP) that helps in strengthening of the muscles and ensures proper muscle and body growth.